ADRENAL FATIGUE RELIEF DIET COOKBOOK

Fuel Your Body with Wholesome and Nutritious Meals

By

Linda Enders

TABLE OF CONTENTS

INTRODUCTION

What is Adrenal Fatigue?

The adrenal glands, which are placed on top of the kidneys, are essential in controlling the body's response to stress. These little but potent glands generate hormones such as cortisol, adrenaline, and norepinephrine, which aid in the management of physical, emotional, and mental stressors.

Adrenal tiredness is a disorder in which the adrenal glands do not function properly. It is also known as hypoadrenia or adrenal insufficiency. This means that hormone synthesis, notably cortisol production, is lowered, resulting in a variety of symptoms that can have an impact on overall health and well-being.

Adrenal fatigue is a controversial topic in the medical community, with some experts disputing its existence as a medical condition. However, many alternative health practitioners believe that adrenal fatigue is a real and common problem, particularly in individuals who lead high-stress lifestyles or have experienced chronic stress.

Symptoms of Adrenal Fatigue

The symptoms of adrenal fatigue can be vague and non-specific, making it challenging to diagnose. However, some of the most common symptoms include:

- Fatigue and low energy levels
- Difficulty waking up in the morning, even after a full night's sleep
- Cravings for sweet or salty foods
- Difficulty handling stress and feeling overwhelmed
- Brain fog and difficulty concentrating
- Decreased sex drive
- Muscle weakness and aches
- Insomnia or disrupted sleep patterns
- Low blood pressure

Causes of Adrenal Fatigue

Adrenal fatigue is thought to be caused by chronic stress, which can be physical, emotional, or mental. Prolonged stress can overtax the adrenal glands, leading to reduced cortisol production and a range of symptoms.

Some of the most common causes of stress that can lead to adrenal fatigue include:

- Work-related stress and long working hours
- Relationship stress or difficulties
- Financial stress
- Chronic illness or injury
- Lack of sleep or disrupted sleep patterns
- Poor diet and nutritional deficiencies
- Exposure to environmental toxins and pollution

Diagnosing Adrenal Fatigue

Adrenal fatigue is not a recognized medical condition, and there is no definitive test for it. However, some alternative health practitioners use a combination of symptom questionnaires, cortisol testing, and blood tests to diagnose adrenal fatigue.

Treatment for Adrenal Fatigue

Adrenal exhaustion treatment often entails lifestyle adjustments such as stress reduction, dietary changes, and supplements. The following are some of the most successful ways for treating adrenal fatigue:

- Meditation, yoga, and deep breathing exercises are all stress-reduction practices.
- A nutrient-dense diet rich in fresh fruits and vegetables, healthy fats, and lean protein sources.
- Avoiding caffeine and alcohol, both of which can cause adrenal gland stress.
- Vitamin and mineral supplements, such as vitamin C, B vitamins, and magnesium
- Getting enough sleep and keeping good sleeping habits

In summary, adrenal fatigue is a disorder in which the adrenal glands do not operate properly, resulting in a variety of symptoms that can have an impact on general health and well-being. Although it is not recognized as a medical ailment by the conventional medical profession, many alternative health practitioners think that adrenal exhaustion is a real and prevalent problem, especially in people who live high-stress lives or have undergone chronic stress. Adrenal exhaustion treatment often entails lifestyle adjustments such as stress reduction, dietary changes, and supplements.

How Diet Can Help Relieve Adrenal Fatigue Symptoms

Our diet can have a big impact on our adrenal function and overall well-being. A healthy and balanced diet can help to nourish the adrenal glands, increase energy, and alleviate symptoms of adrenal fatigue. This chapter will go through how particular dietary adjustments can help alleviate the symptoms of adrenal fatigue.

Adrenal-Friendly Foods

Adrenal fatigue is frequently connected with dietary deficits, thus eating a nutrient-dense diet is critical to supporting the adrenal glands. The following are some of the most critical nutrients for adrenal health:

Vitamin C: This nutrient is essential for the production of cortisol, the primary stress hormone. Citrus fruits, berries, kiwi, broccoli, and bell peppers are excellent sources of vitamin C.

B Vitamins: The B vitamins, including B6, B12, and folate, are critical for energy production and stress management. Meat, fish, eggs, leafy greens, and whole grains are all good sources of B vitamins.

Magnesium: This mineral is necessary for muscle relaxation, stress management, and energy production. Magnesium-rich foods include leafy greens, nuts and seeds, and whole grains.

In addition to these nutrients, it is critical to have a well-balanced diet rich in fresh fruits and vegetables, healthy fats, and lean protein sources. These foods supply the energy and nutrients required to maintain general health and well-being.

Foods to Avoid or Limit

Some foods can aggravate the symptoms of adrenal exhaustion and should be avoided or minimized. These are some examples:

Caffeine: Caffeine can increase cortisol production, leading to further stress on the adrenal glands. Caffeine should be avoided or consumed in minimal amounts in the morning.

Sugar: Excessive sugar consumption can cause blood sugar abnormalities, which can stress the adrenal glands. It's recommended to minimize your sugar intake and use natural sweeteners like honey or maple syrup sparingly.

Processed Foods: Processed foods can contain excessive levels of refined carbs, bad fats, and additives, all of which can stress the adrenal glands. Whenever possible, pick entire, unprocessed meals.

Shopping and Meal Planning Suggestions

Meal planning and preparation in advance can make eating a healthy and balanced diet easier. Some shopping and meal planning suggestions for adrenal fatigue alleviation include:

Buy fresh veggies and lean protein sources like grass-fed beef, free-range poultry, and wild-caught fish.

Plan meals that include nutrient-dense foods like leafy greens, berries, nuts and seeds, and healthy fats.

Prepare meals ahead of time and keep them in the fridge or freezer for quick and easy meals throughout the week.

To assist maintain energy levels throughout the day, choose adrenal-friendly snacks such as fresh fruit, nuts, and seed butter.

In conclusion, a healthy and balanced diet helps promote adrenal health and alleviate symptoms of adrenal fatigue. Eating nutrient-dense foods, limiting or eliminating caffeine, sugar, and processed foods, and planning meals ahead of time can all help ease symptoms of adrenal fatigue. Individuals suffering from adrenal fatigue can improve their general health and well-being by making dietary modifications.

How This Cookbook Can Help You

This Adrenal Fatigue Relief Diet Cookbook is intended to assist those suffering from adrenal fatigue in making dietary modifications that will improve their symptoms and general health. This chapter will go over how this cookbook can assist you in managing your adrenal exhaustion.

Recipes Designed for Adrenal-Friendly Eating

This cookbook's recipes are all intended to enhance adrenal health and alleviate symptoms of adrenal exhaustion. They're packed with nutrients including fresh fruits and veggies, healthy fats, and lean protein sources. These meals are also free of caffeine, refined sugar, and processed foods, which can aggravate the symptoms of adrenal exhaustion.

Adrenal Health Support

This cookbook offers advice and information on how to improve adrenal health through nutrition. It contains information on the nutrients required to maintain adrenal function, as well as suggestions on how to shop, plan, and prepare meals for adrenal fatigue alleviation. The cookbook also includes tips on how to deal with stress and enhance overall well-being.

Reduced Symptoms and Increased Energy

Individuals suffering from adrenal fatigue can increase their energy levels and lessen symptoms such as exhaustion, brain fog, and mood swings by following the recipes and meal plans in this cookbook. Nutrient-dense foods and balanced meals can assist maintain adrenal function while also promoting general health and well-being.

In conclusion, this Adrenal Fatigue Relief Diet Cookbook can assist persons suffering from adrenal fatigue in making dietary modifications that benefit their overall health and well-being. Individuals can control their symptoms and enhance their quality of life by using the recipes, food plans, and advice on adrenal health. Individuals may take control of their health and start feeling better now by utilizing this cookbook as a guide.

BREAKFAST RECIPES

Breakfasts That Energize and Sustain

Green Smoothie Bowl with Berries and Nuts

Ingredients:

- 1 cup mixed frozen berries
- 1 frozen banana
- 1 cup spinach, fresh
- 1/2 cup almond milk
- 1 tbsp. honey
- 1 tbsp. chia seeds
- 1/4 cup chopped mixed nuts

Instructions:

1. Blend together the frozen berries, frozen banana, fresh spinach, almond milk, honey, and chia seeds in a blender.
2. On high, blend until smooth and creamy.
3. Pour the smoothie into a bowl and top with chopped mixed nuts.
4. Serve right away and enjoy!

Sweet Potato and Turkey Sausage Hash

Ingredients:

- 1 large sweet potato, peeled and cubed
- 1 small onion, chopped
- 2 cloves garlic, minced
- 2 turkey sausages, sliced
- 1 tbsp. olive oil
- 1/2 tsp. smoked paprika
- 1/4 tsp. cumin
- Salt and black pepper, to taste
- Fresh parsley, chopped (for garnish)

Instructions:

1. Warm the olive oil in a large skillet over medium heat.
2. Sauté the chopped onion and minced garlic for 2-3 minutes, or until fragrant.
3. Sauté the diced sweet potato in the skillet for 8-10 minutes, or until soft and tender.
4. Sauté the sliced turkey sausage, smoked paprika, cumin, salt, and black pepper in the skillet for 5 minutes, or until the sausage is fully cooked.

5. Remove the skillet from the heat and top with fresh parsley.

6. Serve right away and enjoy!

Baked Eggs with Spinach and Feta

Ingredients:

- 4 eggs
- 1/2 cup chopped fresh spinach
- 1/4 cup feta cheese, crumbled
- 2 tbsp. olive oil
- Salt and black pepper, to taste

Instructions:

1. Preheat the oven to 375 degrees Fahrenheit (190 degrees Celsius).

2. Warm the olive oil in a large oven-safe skillet over medium heat.

3. Sauté the chopped spinach in the skillet for 2-3 minutes, or until wilted.

4. Pour the eggs into the skillet over the sautéed spinach.

5. Season the eggs with salt and black pepper and top with crumbled feta cheese.

6. Bake for 8-10 minutes, or until the eggs are set and the cheese is melted, in a preheated oven.

7. Remove the pan from the oven and set aside for a few minutes to cool.

8. Serve the baked eggs immediately and enjoy!

Breakfast Bowl with Quinoa, Fresh Fruit, and Almonds

Ingredients:

- 1 cup quinoa, cooked
- 1/2 cup mixed fresh fruit (such as berries, kiwi, or banana)
- 2 tbsp. slivered almonds
- 1 tbsp. honey
- 1/4 tsp. cinnamon

Instructions:

1. In a mixing bowl, combine the cooked quinoa, fresh fruit, and slivered almonds.

2. Drizzle honey over the top and sprinkle with cinnamon.

3. Serve right away and enjoy!

Toast with avocado, poached eggs, and tomato

Ingredients:

- 2 whole-grain bread slices, toasted
- 1 ripe avocado, mashed
- 2 eggs, poached
- 1 medium tomato, sliced
- Salt and black pepper to taste
- Fresh parsley, chopped (for garnish)

Instructions:

1. Toast the bread slices till golden brown in a toaster or on a grill.
2. Evenly spread the mashed avocado across the toasted bread slices.
3. Add a poached egg and sliced tomato to each slice of avocado toast.
4. To taste, season with salt and black pepper.
5. Garnish with fresh parsley, if desired.
6. Serve right away and enjoy!

Omelet with Veggies, Goat Cheese, and Herbs

Ingredients:

- 3 eggs
- 1/4 cup mixed veggies
- 1 oz. crumbled goat cheese
- 1 tbsp. olive oil
- Salt and black pepper, to taste
- Fresh herbs (parsley or chives, for example), chopped (for garnish)

Instructions:

1. Whisk the eggs with salt and black pepper in a small bowl.
2. Heat the olive oil in a nonstick skillet over medium heat.
3. Sauté the mixed vegetables in the skillet for 2-3 minutes, or until soft and tender.
4. Pour the whisked eggs into the skillet with the sautéed vegetables and simmer until the eggs begin to set.
5. Sprinkle the crumbled goat cheese over the omelet and cook until the cheese melts and the eggs are fully cooked.

6. Remove the skillet from the heat and top with fresh herbs.

7. Serve the vegetable omelet immediately and enjoy!

Nutrient-Dense Smoothies

Pineapple and Spinach Tropical Green Smoothie

Ingredients:

- 1 cup fresh pineapple chunks
- 1 cup fresh spinach leaves
- 1 banana, medium ripe
- 1/2 cup almond milk, unsweetened
- 1/2 cup Greek yogurt, plain
- 1 tbsp. honey (optional)

Instructions:

1. In a blender, combine the fresh pineapple pieces, fresh spinach leaves, ripe banana, unsweetened almond milk, and plain Greek yogurt.

2. On high speed, combine the ingredients until smooth and creamy.

3. Taste the smoothie and adjust the sweetness with honey if necessary.

4. Serve the tropical green smoothie immediately in a glass.

Chocolate Banana Smoothie with Almond Butter and Cacao Powder

Ingredients:

- 1 banana, ripe
- 1 tbsp. almond butter
- 1 tbsp. cacao powder
- 1 cup unsweetened almond milk
- 1/2 tsp. vanilla extract
- 1/2 cup cubed ice

Instructions:

1. In a blender, combine the ripe banana, almond butter, cacao powder, unsweetened almond milk, vanilla extract, and ice cubes.
2. On high speed, combine the ingredients until smooth and creamy.
3. Serve the chocolate banana smoothie immediately in a glass.

Berry Blast Smoothie with Mixed Berries and Greek Yogurt

Ingredients:

- 1 cup frozen mixed berries (strawberries, raspberries, and blueberries)
- 1/2 cup Greek yogurt, plain
- 1/2 cup almond milk, unsweetened
- 1 tbsp. honey (optional)

Instructions:

1. In a blender, combine the frozen mixed berries, plain Greek yogurt, and unsweetened almond milk.
2. On high speed, combine the ingredients until smooth and creamy.
3. Taste the smoothie and adjust the sweetness with honey if necessary.
4. Serve the berry blast smoothie immediately in a glass.

Ginger and Turmeric Mango Turmeric Smoothie

Ingredients:

- 1 cup mango chunks, frozen
- 1 banana
- 1/2 cup Greek yogurt, plain
- 1/2 cup almond milk, unsweetened
- 1 tsp. grated ginger
- 1/2 tsp. ground turmeric
- 1 tbsp. honey (optional)

Instructions:

1. In a blender, combine the frozen mango chunks, banana, plain Greek yogurt, unsweetened almond milk, grated ginger, and crushed turmeric.
2. On high speed, combine the ingredients until smooth and creamy.
3. Taste the smoothie and adjust the sweetness with honey if necessary.
4. Serve the mango turmeric smoothie right away in a glass.

Green Tea Smoothie with Matcha and Coconut Milk

Ingredients:

- 1 cup unsweetened coconut milk
- 1 tsp. matcha green tea powder
- 1 banana
- 1/2 cup fresh spinach leaves
- 1/2 cup frozen pineapple chunks
- 1 tbsp. honey (optional)

Instructions:

1. In a blender, combine the unsweetened coconut milk, matcha green tea powder, banana, fresh spinach leaves, frozen pineapple pieces, and honey (if using).
2. On high speed, combine the ingredients until smooth and creamy.
3. Serve the green tea smoothie immediately in a glass.

Maple Cinnamon Oatmeal Bowl with Walnuts and Raisins

Ingredients:

- 1/2 cup rolled oats
- 1 cup of water
- 1/4 tsp. cinnamon
- 1 tbsp. maple syrup
- 2 tbsp. chopped walnuts
- 2 tbsp. raisins

Instructions:

1. Combine the rolled oats, water, and cinnamon in a small saucepan.
2. Bring the mixture to a boil, stirring occasionally, over medium-high heat.
3. Reduce the heat to low and continue to cook the oats for 5-7 minutes or until the desired thickness is reached.
4. Take the oats from the heat and add the maple syrup.

5. Place the oatmeal in a bowl and top with the walnuts and raisins.

6. Warm the maple cinnamon oatmeal bowl before serving.

Banana Nut Oatmeal Bowl with Almond Milk and Chia Seeds

Ingredients:

- 1/2 cup rolled oats
- 1 cup almond milk, unsweetened
- 1 mashed banana
- 1 tbsp. chia seeds
- 2 tbsp. nuts (almonds, pecans, or walnuts) chopped
- 1 tbsp. honey (optional)

Instructions:

1. Combine the rolled oats and unsweetened almond milk in a small saucepan.

2. Bring the mixture to a boil, stirring occasionally, over medium-high heat.

3. Reduce the heat to low and continue to cook the oats for 5-7 minutes or until the desired thickness is reached.

4. Take the oats off the stove and add the mashed banana and chia seeds.

5. Top the oats with the chopped nuts and honey (if using) and serve.

6. Serve the banana nut oatmeal bowl immediately.

Apple Cinnamon Oatmeal Bowl with Greek Yogurt and Honey

Ingredients:

- 1/2 cup rolled oats
- 1 cup of water
- 1/2 grated apple
- 1/4 tsp. cinnamon
- 1/4 cup plain Greek yogurt
- 1 tbsp. honey
- 1 tbsp. (optional) chopped nuts

Instructions:

1. Combine the rolled oats, water, grated apple, and cinnamon in a small saucepan.

2. Bring the mixture to a boil, stirring occasionally, over medium-high heat.

3. Reduce the heat to low and continue to cook the oats for 5-7 minutes or until the desired thickness is reached.

4. Remove the oatmeal from the heat and whisk in the honey and plain Greek yogurt.

5. Place the oatmeal in a bowl and sprinkle with chopped nuts, if using.

6. Serve the warm apple cinnamon oatmeal bowl.

Energizing Egg Dishes

Spinach and Mushroom Frittata with Feta Cheese:

Ingredients:

- 6 large eggs
- 1/2 cup spinach, chopped
- 1/2 cup mushrooms, sliced
- 1/4 cup feta cheese, crumbled
- 2 tbsp. olive oil
- Salt and pepper to taste

Instructions:

1. Preheat the oven to 375 degrees Fahrenheit.

2. Whisk together the eggs, salt, and pepper in a large mixing basin.

3. In an oven-safe skillet, heat the olive oil over medium heat.

4. Cook until the spinach and mushrooms are wilted, about 5 minutes.

5. Pour the egg mixture over the veggies and simmer for 5 minutes, or until the edges begin to firm.

6. Spread feta cheese on top of the frittata.

7. Bake the skillet for 10-12 minutes, or until the middle is set and the top is golden brown.

8. Remove from the oven and set aside for 5 minutes to cool.

9. Serve heated, sliced.

Veggie and Cheese Omelet with Whole Grain Toast:

Ingredients:

- 2 large eggs
- 1/4 cup bell peppers, chopped
- 1/4 cup diced onion
- 1/4 cup shredded cheddar

- 1 tablespoon olive oil
- Salt and pepper to taste
- 1 whole grain bread piece

Instructions:

1. Beat the eggs in a small bowl and season with salt and pepper.
2. In a nonstick skillet over medium heat, heat the olive oil.
3. Sauté the bell peppers and onions for 3-4 minutes, or until tender.
4. Pour the eggs into the skillet and swirl them around to coat the bottom.
5. Cook for about 2-3 minutes, or until the eggs begin to set.
6. One half of the omelet should be topped with shredded cheese.
7. Fold the other half of the omelet over the cheese with a spatula and cook for another 1-2 minutes, or until the cheese is melted and the eggs are cooked through.
8. Serve immediately with whole grain bread.

Scrambled Eggs with Smoked Salmon and Dill:

Ingredients:

- 2 large eggs
- 1 oz. smoked salmon, chopped
- 1 tbsp. chopped fresh dill
- 1 tbsp. unsalted butter
- Salt and pepper to taste

Instructions:

1. Whisk together the eggs, salt, and pepper in a small bowl.
2. In a nonstick skillet over medium heat, melt the butter.
3. Cook, stirring regularly, until the eggs begin to set, about 1-2 minutes.
4. Cook for another 1-2 minutes, or until the eggs are fully cooked, with the smoked salmon and dill.
5. Serve immediately.

LUNCH RECIPES

Lunches That Keep You Going

Grilled Chicken and Veggie Skewers with Quinoa Salad

Ingredients:

- 1 lb. chicken breast, cut into cubes
- 2 sliced zucchinis
- 1 sliced red bell pepper
- 1 sliced yellow bell pepper
- 1 sliced onion
- 1 tbsp. olive oil
- Salt and pepper to taste
- 1 cup quinoa, cooked
- 1/2 cup cherry tomatoes, halved
- 1/4 cup fresh parsley, chopped
- 2 tbsp. lemon juice
- 1 tbsp. olive oil

Instructions:

1. Preheat the grill to medium-high.

2. Thread skewers with chicken, zucchini, red bell pepper, yellow bell pepper, and onion.

3. Brush olive oil on skewers and season with salt and pepper.

4. Grill the skewers for 10-12 minutes, flipping occasionally, until the chicken is thoroughly cooked.

5. Combine cooked quinoa, cherry tomatoes, parsley, lemon juice, and olive oil in a medium mixing bowl. Season to taste with salt and pepper.

6. Skewers should be served with quinoa salad on the side.

Rainbow Veggie Wrap with Hummus and Avocado

Ingredients:

- 4 large collard green leaves
- 1/2 cup hummus
- 1 avocado, sliced
- 1 red bell pepper, sliced
- 1 yellow bell pepper, sliced
- 1 carrot, grated
- 1/4 red cabbage, sliced

- Season with salt and pepper to taste.

Instructions:

1. A large pot of water should be brought to a boil. Blanch collard green leaves for 30 seconds in boiling water, then drain and pat dry with paper towels.
2. Distribute hummus evenly across each collard green leaf.
3. On top of the hummus, layer avocado, red bell pepper, yellow bell pepper, grated carrot, and red cabbage.
4. Season to taste with salt and pepper.
5. Form wraps by tightly rolling collard green leaves around the filling.
6. Serve the wraps cut in half.

Lentil and Vegetable Soup with Whole Grain Bread

Ingredients:

- 1 cup dried green lentils, rinsed and drained
- 1 onion, chopped
- 2 carrots, chopped
- 2 stalks celery, chopped

- 2 garlic cloves, minced
- 6 cups vegetable broth (low sodium)
- 1 tomato can, diced
- 1 tsp. dried thyme
- Salt and pepper to taste
- 4 slices toasted whole grain bread
- 1/4 cup grated Parmesan cheese

Instructions:

1. Combine lentils, onion, carrots, celery, garlic, vegetable broth, chopped tomatoes, thyme, salt, and pepper in a large pot.

2. Bring the mixture to a boil, then reduce to a low heat and cook for 25-30 minutes, or until the lentils are cooked.

3. Place a slice of toasted whole grain bread on top of each cup of soup.

4. Each bowl should be topped with grated Parmesan cheese.

5. Serve immediately.

Chicken and Quinoa Salad with Mixed Greens and Lemon Vinaigrette:

Ingredients:

- 1 cup quinoa, cooked
- 2 cups greens, mixed
- 1 cup shredded cooked chicken
- 1/2 cup halved cherry tomatoes
- 1/4 cup chopped red onion
- 1/4 cup cucumber, chopped
- 14 cup diced bell pepper
- 1/4 cup feta cheese, crumbled
- 2 tbsp. of lemon juice
- 1 tablespoon extra-virgin olive oil
- 1 tsp. Dijon mustard
- Season with salt and pepper to taste.

Instructions:

1. Combine the cooked quinoa, mixed greens, chicken, cherry tomatoes, red onion, cucumber, and bell pepper in a large mixing bowl.

2. Whisk together the lemon juice, olive oil, Dijon mustard, salt, and pepper in a small bowl.

3. Toss the salad with the dressing to mix.

4. Serve with crumbled feta cheese on top.

Sweet Potato and Kale Soup with Chickpeas and Turmeric:

Ingredients:

- 1 tablespoon extra-virgin olive oil
- 1 chopped onion
- 2 minced garlic cloves
- 1 peeled and sliced sweet potato
- 1 can drained and washed chickpeas
- 4 cups veggie broth
- 2 cups kale, chopped
- 1 tablespoon turmeric
- Season with salt and pepper to taste.

Instructions:

1. Warm the olive oil in a big pot over medium heat. Sauté the onion and garlic for 2-3 minutes or until the onion is transparent.

2. Pour in the sweet potato, chickpeas, and vegetable broth. Bring to a boil, then reduce to a low heat and continue to cook for 20-25 minutes or until the sweet potato is cooked.

3. Stir in the kale and turmeric until the kale is completely wilted.

4. Season to taste with salt and pepper.

5. Serve immediately with whole grain toast.

Spinach and Quinoa Salad with Roasted Vegetables and Feta Cheese:

Ingredients:

- 1 cup quinoa, cooked
- 2 cups fresh baby spinach
- 1/2 cup halved cherry tomatoes
- 1/2 cup roasted veggies (zucchini, bell peppers, eggplant, etc.)
- 1/4 cup feta cheese, crumbled
- 2 tbsp. of olive oil
- 1 tbsp. balsamic vinegar
- Season with salt and pepper to taste.

Instructions:

1. Combine the cooked quinoa, baby spinach, cherry tomatoes, and roasted veggies in a large mixing basin.
2. In a small mixing bowl, combine the olive oil, balsamic vinegar, salt, and pepper.
3. Toss the salad with the dressing to mix.
4. Serve with crumbled feta cheese on top.

Satisfying Sandwiches and Wraps

Grilled Chicken and Veggie Wrap with Tzatziki Sauce

Ingredients:

- 1 whole-wheat wrap, large
- 4 oz. grilled chicken breast, sliced
- 1 cup of mixed greens
- 1/4 cup red onion, sliced
- 1/4 cup cucumber, sliced
- 1/4 cup bell pepper, sliced
- 2 tbsp. tzatziki sauce

Instructions:

1. Spread the tzatziki sauce over the wrap and place it on a flat surface.

2. On top of the sauce, layer the sliced chicken breast, mixed greens, red onion, cucumber, and bell pepper.

3. Wrap it tightly and cut it in half diagonally.

Sandwich of turkey and avocado with sprouts and mustard

Ingredients:

- 2 slices whole-grain bread
- 4 oz. turkey breast
- 1/4 sliced avocado
- 1/4 cup sprouted alfalfa
- 1 tablespoon Dijon mustard

Instructions:

1. Toast the slices of bread till golden brown.

2. On one slice of bread, spread the Dijon mustard.

3. On top of the mustard, layer the turkey breast, avocado slices, and alfalfa sprouts.

4. Place the other slice of bread on top.

Wrap with Hummus, Roasted Red Peppers, and Spinach

Ingredients:

- 1 whole-wheat wrap, large
- 1/4 cup hummus
- 1/4 cup sliced roasted red peppers
- 1 cup fresh baby spinach leaves
- 1/4 cup cucumber, sliced
- 1/4 cup carrot, sliced

Instructions:

1. Spread the hummus on top of the wrap.
2. On top of the hummus, arrange the roasted red peppers, baby spinach leaves, sliced cucumber, and sliced carrot.
3. Wrap it tightly and cut it in half diagonally.

Burrito with black beans and sweet potatoes, brown rice, and salsa.

Ingredients:

- 1 large sweet potato, peeled and diced
- 1 tablespoon extra-virgin olive oil
- 1 tsp. chili powder
- 1/2 teaspoon cumin
- paprika, 1/2 teaspoon
- Salt and pepper to taste
- 1 can black beans, drained and rinsed
- 1 cup brown rice, cooked
- 4 whole wheat tortillas
- Salsa to serve

Instructions:

1. Preheat the oven to 400 degrees Fahrenheit (200 degrees Celsius).
2. Toss the diced sweet potato with the olive oil, chili powder, cumin, paprika, salt, and pepper in a mixing bowl until equally coated.

3. Roast the sweet potatoes in a single layer on a baking sheet for 20-25 minutes, or until soft and lightly browned.

4. Heat the black beans in a small saucepan over medium heat until heated through.

5. Warm the tortillas for a few minutes in the oven, or until soft and malleable.

6. Spread a quarter of the brown rice in the center of each tortilla, leaving about an inch border around the borders.

7. Place a quarter of the roasted sweet potatoes and black beans on top of each tortilla.

8. Tuck the edges in as you roll the tortillas securely.

9. If desired, serve with salsa on the side.

Mediterranean Quinoa Bowl with Hummus, Roasted Vegetables, and Feta Cheese

Ingredients:

- 1 cup quinoa, cooked
- 1 hummus cup
- 1 cup roasted veggies (bell peppers, zucchini, eggplant, etc.)
- 2 tablespoons crumbled feta cheese
- chopped fresh parsley
- Salt and pepper to taste

Instructions:

1. Cook the quinoa according to the package directions and set it aside.
2. Cook until the vegetables are soft and slightly browned in the oven or on the grill.
3. Place cooked quinoa at the bottom of the bowl, followed by roasted vegetables and hummus on top.
4. Top with crumbled feta cheese and minced parsley.
5. Season to taste with salt and pepper.

Roasted Vegetable and Brown Rice Bowl with Avocado and Tahini Dressing

Ingredients:

- 1 cup brown rice, cooked
- 1 cup roasted veggies (sweet potatoes, Brussels sprouts, carrots, etc.)
- 1/2 sliced avocado
- 2 tbsp. tahini
- 1 tablespoon lemon juice
- 1 minced garlic clove
- Water, as needed
- Season with salt and pepper to taste.

Instructions:

1. Brown rice should be cooked according to package directions and set aside.
2. Cook until the vegetables are soft and slightly browned in the oven or on the grill.
3. Whisk together tahini, lemon juice, garlic, and enough water to produce a pourable dressing in a small bowl.
4. Place cooked brown rice in the bottom of the bowl, followed by roasted vegetables and sliced avocado.

5. Drizzle the tahini dressing on top of the bowl.

6. Season to taste with salt and pepper.

Sweet Potato and Black Bean Bowl with Quinoa and Cilantro-Lime Dressing

Ingredients:

- 1 cup quinoa, cooked
- 1 cup sweet potatoes, roasted
- 1 cup black beans, drained and rinsed
- 1/4 cup chopped red onion
- 1/4 cup fresh cilantro, chopped
- 1 lime, juiced
- 1 tbsp. olive oil
- Salt and pepper to taste

Instructions

1. Cook the quinoa according to the package directions and set it aside.

2. Roast sweet potatoes till crisp and slightly browned in the oven or on the grill.

3. To make the dressing, whisk together lime juice, olive oil, salt, and pepper in a small bowl.

4. Place cooked quinoa at the bottom of the bowl, followed by roasted sweet potatoes, black beans, red onion, and cilantro on top.

5. Drizzle the cilantro-lime dressing on top of the salad.

6. Season to taste with salt and pepper.

DINNER RECIPES

Dinners That Restore and Recharge

Grilled Salmon with Roasted Asparagus and Quinoa

Ingredients:

- 4 salmon fillets
- 1 bunch of asparagus
- 1 cup quinoa
- 2 cups water or broth
- 2 tbsp. of olive oil
- Salt and pepper, to taste

Instructions:

1. Preheat the oven to 400 degrees Fahrenheit.

2. Rinse the quinoa and place it in a pot with water or broth to cook. Bring to a boil, then reduce to a low heat and continue to cook for 15-20 minutes or until the liquid is absorbed and the quinoa is cooked.

3. Rinse the asparagus and snap off the rough ends. Place them on a baking pan and season with salt and pepper. Roast for 10-15 minutes, or until tender.

4. Preheat a grill pan or an outdoor grill to medium-high. Season the salmon fillets with salt and pepper before grilling them. Cook for 3-4 minutes per side, or until thoroughly done.

5. Serve the salmon with quinoa and roasted asparagus on the side.

Turkey and Sweet Potato Chili with Mixed Greens Salad

Ingredients:

- 1 pound turkey ground
- 2 peeled and sliced sweet potatoes
- 1 can drained and rinsed black beans
- 1 tomato can, diced
- 1 diced onion
- 2 minced garlic cloves
- 2 tablespoons chili powder
- 1 tablespoon cumin
- Salt and pepper to taste
- 4 cups greens, mixed
- 1 tbsp. olive oil
- 2 tbsp. apple cider vinegar
- 1 tbsp. honey

Instructions:

1. Warm up a big saucepan over medium-high heat. Cook, breaking up the ground turkey with a spoon, until browned and cooked through.

2. In the pot, combine the sweet potatoes, black beans, chopped tomatoes, onion, garlic, chili powder, cumin, salt, and pepper. To blend, stir everything together thoroughly.

3. Bring the chili to a boil, then reduce to a low heat and simmer for 30 minutes, or until the sweet potatoes are soft and the flavors have merged.

4. To make the dressing, whisk together the olive oil, apple cider vinegar, honey, salt, and pepper in a small bowl.

5. Serve the chili with a dish of vinaigrette-dressed mixed greens.

Baked Chicken with Roasted Root Vegetables and Brown Rice

Ingredients:

- 4 skinless, boneless chicken breasts
- 1 large peeled and cut into 1-inch pieces sweet potato
- 2 peeled and cut into 1-inch pieces parsnips
- 2 peeled and sliced carrots into 1-inch chunks
- 1 red onion, peeled and cut into wedges
- 2 tbsp. olive oil
- Salt and black pepper
- 1 tsp. garlic powder
- 1 teaspoon thyme dried
- 1 cup brown rice, cooked according to package instructions

Instructions:

1. Preheat the oven to 400 degrees Fahrenheit.
2. Combine the sweet potato, parsnips, carrots, and red onion in a large mixing bowl. Season with salt, black pepper, garlic powder, and thyme and drizzle with olive oil. To coat, toss with a fork.

3. Arrange the vegetables in a single layer on a baking sheet. On top of the vegetables, place the chicken breasts. Season the chicken with black pepper and salt.

4. Bake for 25-30 minutes, or until the chicken is thoroughly cooked and the vegetables are soft.

5. Serve alongside brown rice.

Lentil and Vegetable Stir-Fry with Brown Rice Noodles

Ingredients:

- 8 oz. brown rice noodles
- 1 tablespoon extra-virgin olive oil
- 1 onion, chopped
- 2 garlic cloves, minced
- 1 red bell pepper, sliced
- 1 yellow bell pepper, sliced
- 2 cups sliced mushrooms
- 1 can lentils, drained and rinsed
- 2 tbsp. of soy sauce
- 1 tablespoon vinegar (rice)
- 1 tablespoon honey
- 1 teaspoon fresh ginger, grated

- 1/4 teaspoon crushed red pepper flakes
- Salt and black pepper
- Chopped fresh cilantro for garnish

Instructions:

1. Brown rice noodles should be cooked according to package directions. Set aside after draining.
2. In a large skillet over medium-high heat, heat the olive oil. Sauté the onion and garlic for 2-3 minutes, or until softened.
3. Sauté the bell peppers and mushrooms in the skillet for 5-7 minutes, or until soft.
4. Combine the lentils, soy sauce, rice vinegar, honey, ginger, red pepper flakes, salt, and black pepper in a large mixing bowl. Cook for 2-3 minutes, or until the lentils are well heated.
5. Toss the cooked brown rice noodles into the skillet to incorporate.
6. Garnish with chopped cilantro and serve hot.

Slow-Cooked Beef Stew with Root Vegetables and Herbs

Ingredients:

- 2 lbs. beef stew meat, cut into 1-inch pieces
- 2 tablespoons olive oil
- 1 onion, chopped
- 3 cloves garlic, minced
- 3 cups beef broth
- 1 cup red wine
- 2 carrots, peeled and chopped
- 2 parsnips, peeled and chopped
- 2 potatoes, peeled and chopped
- 2 tablespoons tomato paste
- 1 teaspoon dried thyme
- 1 teaspoon dried rosemary
- Salt and pepper to taste

Directions:

1. In a large skillet over medium-high heat, heat the olive oil.

2. Brown the beef stew flesh on all sides, about 5-7 minutes.

3. Place the steak in a slow cooker.

4. Sauté the onion and garlic in the skillet for 3-5 minutes, or until softened.

5. In the slow cooker, combine the beef broth, red wine, carrots, parsnips, potatoes, tomato paste, thyme, and rosemary.

6. Season with salt and pepper and stir to mix.

7. Cook for 6-8 hours on low, or until the beef is cooked.

8. Serve immediately and enjoy.

Grilled Chicken with Sweet Potato Mash and Steamed Broccoli

Ingredients:

- 4 skinless, boneless chicken breasts
- 1 tablespoon extra-virgin olive oil
- 1 teaspoon garlic powder
- 1 teaspoon dried thyme
- Salt and pepper to taste

- 2 sweet potatoes, peeled and chopped
- 1/4 cup unsweetened almond milk
- 2 tablespoons butter
- 2 cups broccoli florets

Directions:

1. Preheat the grill to medium-high temperature.
2. Olive oil, garlic powder, thyme, salt, and pepper season the chicken breasts.
3. Grill the chicken for 6-8 minutes per side, or until done.
4. Cook the sweet potatoes in a pot of water until soft, about 10-12 minutes, while the chicken is grilling.
5. Mash the sweet potatoes with almond milk and butter.
6. Season to taste with salt and pepper.
7. In a steamer basket, cook the broccoli florets until tender, about 5-7 minutes.
8. On the side, serve the grilled chicken with a scoop of sweet potato mash and steamed broccoli.
9. Enjoy!

Shepherd's Pie with Cauliflower Mash and Ground Turkey

Ingredients:

- 1 lb. ground turkey
- 1 onion, chopped
- 2 cloves garlic, minced
- 2 cups mixed veggies (carrots, peas, corn, etc.)
- 1 cup chicken or beef broth
- 2 tablespoons tomato paste
- 1 teaspoon dried thyme
- Salt and pepper, to taste
- 1 sliced head cauliflower 2 tbsp. butter
- 1/4 cup milk

Instructions:

1. Preheat the oven to 375 degrees Fahrenheit.
2. Cook ground turkey in a large skillet over medium heat until browned and no longer pink, about 10 minutes. Remove any extra fat.
3. Cook for 2-3 minutes or until the onion and garlic is softened.
4. Combine the vegetables, chicken or beef broth, tomato paste, dried thyme, salt, and pepper in a

mixing bowl. Stir everything together and cook for 10 minutes.

5. Meanwhile, simmer chopped cauliflower in a large saucepan of boiling water until soft, about 10 minutes.

6. Return the cauliflower to the pot after draining. Mash in the butter, milk, salt, and pepper until smooth.

7. Fill a baking dish halfway with the turkey and vegetable mixture. Cover the top of the mixture with the mashed cauliflower.

8. 25-30 minutes, or until the top is golden brown and the filling is bubbling.

Stir-Fry Beef and Vegetables with Brown Rice

Ingredients:

- 1 lb. beef sirloin, sliced into thin strips
- 2 tablespoons olive oil
- 2 minced garlic cloves
- 1 sliced onion
- 2 cups mixed veggies (broccoli, bell peppers, carrots, etc.)
- 1 tablespoon soy sauce

- 2 tablespoons honey
- 1 tablespoon cornstarch
- Salt and pepper, to taste
- 3 cups cooked brown rice

Instructions:

1. Heat the olive oil in a big skillet or wok over high heat.
2. Cook for 2-3 minutes or until the garlic and onion is softened.
3. Cook the sliced beef in the skillet for 2-3 minutes, or until browned.
4. Stir-fry the mixed vegetables in the skillet for 3-4 minutes, or until they are cooked but still crisp.
5. In a small mixing bowl, combine soy sauce, honey, cornstarch, salt, and pepper.
6. Stir the sauce into the skillet to coat the steak and vegetables.
7. Cook for another 2-3 minutes, or until the sauce thickens.
8. Serve immediately with prepared brown rice.

SNACK AND DESSERT RECIPES

Snacks That Fuel and Sustain

Energy Balls with Dates and Almonds

Ingredients:

- 1 cup pitted Medjool dates
- 1 cup raw almonds
- 1/4 tsp. sea salt
- 1 tsp. vanilla extract
- 1/4 cup shredded coconut

Instructions:

1. In a food processor, pulse the dates and almonds until they form a sticky mixture.

2. Add the sea salt, vanilla extract, and shredded coconut, and pulse until everything is well combined.

3. Roll the mixture into small balls, about the size of a golf ball.

4. Store the energy balls in an airtight container in the fridge for up to a week.

Greek Yogurt Parfait with Berries and Granola

Ingredients:

- 1 cup plain Greek yogurt
- 1/2 cup mixed berries (such as blueberries, raspberries, and strawberries)
- 1/4 cup granola
- 1 tbsp. honey

Instructions:

1. In a small bowl, mix together the Greek yogurt and honey.
2. Layer the yogurt mixture, mixed berries, and granola in a glass or jar.
3. Serve immediately or store in the fridge for up to a day.

Baked Apple Chips with Cinnamon

Ingredients:

- 2 apples
- 1 tsp. cinnamon

Instructions:

1. Preheat the oven to 200°F (93°C).

2. Slice the apples thinly (about 1/8 inch thick) and remove the seeds and cores.

3. Arrange the apple slices on a baking sheet lined with parchment paper.

4. Sprinkle cinnamon over the apple slices.

5. Bake for 1-2 hours, or until the apple slices are crispy.

6. Let the apple chips cool completely before storing them in an airtight container.

Chocolate Avocado Pudding

Ingredients:

- 2 ripe avocados
- 1/2 cup unsweetened cocoa powder
- 1/2 cup honey
- 1/4 cup almond milk
- 1 tsp. vanilla extract

Instructions:

1. In a food processor, blend the avocados until they are smooth and creamy.

2. Add the cocoa powder, honey, almond milk, and vanilla extract, and blend until everything is well combined.

3. Spoon the pudding into small bowls or jars and chill in the fridge for at least 1 hour before serving.

Trail Mix with Nuts and Seeds

Ingredients:

- 1 cup mixed nuts (such as almonds, walnuts, and cashews)
- 1/2 cup pumpkin seeds
- 1/2 cup sunflower seeds
- 1/4 cup dried cranberries
- 1/4 cup dark chocolate chips

Instructions:

1. Combine the nuts, seeds, and dried cranberries in a large mixing dish.
2. Mix in the dark chocolate chips once more.
3. For up to a week, store the trail mix in an airtight jar at room temperature.

Acai Berry Smoothie Bowl with Granola and Mixed Berries

Ingredients:

- 1 frozen banana
- 1/2 cup frozen mixed berries
- 1/4 cup unsweetened almond milk
- 1 packet frozen acai
- 1 tbsp. honey
- 1/4 cup granola
- 1/4 cup mixed berries
- 1 tbsp. chia seeds

Instructions:

1. In a blender, combine the frozen banana, mixed berries, almond milk, acai, and honey.
2. Blend until smooth and creamy, scraping down the sides as necessary.
3. Fill a bowl halfway with the smoothie.
4. Sprinkle the granola, mixed berries, and chia seeds on top of the smoothie.
5. Serve right away and enjoy!

Mango and Pineapple Smoothie Bowl with Coconut Flakes and Chia Seeds

Ingredients:

- 1/2 cup frozen mango
- 1/2 cup frozen pineapple
- 1/4 cup unsweetened coconut milk
- 1 tbsp. honey
- 1/4 cup granola
- 1 tbsp. coconut flakes
- 1 tbsp. chia seeds

Instructions:

1. In a blender, combine the frozen mango, pineapple, coconut milk, and honey.
2. Blend until smooth and creamy, scraping down the sides as necessary.
3. Fill a bowl halfway with the smoothie.
4. Sprinkle the granola, coconut flakes, and chia seeds on top of the smoothie.
5. Serve right away and enjoy!

Chocolate Banana Smoothie Bowl with Almond Butter and Cacao Nibs

Ingredients:

- 1 frozen banana
- 1/4 cup unsweetened almond milk
- 1 tbsp. honey
- 1 tbsp. almond butter
- 1 tbsp. cacao powder
- 1/4 cup granola
- 1 tbsp. cacao nibs

Instructions:

1. In a blender, combine the frozen banana, almond milk, honey, almond butter, and cacao powder.
2. Blend until smooth and creamy, scraping down the sides as necessary.
3. Fill a bowl halfway with the smoothie.
4. Sprinkle the granola and cacao nibs on top of the smoothie.
5. Serve right away and enjoy!

Mixed Berry Smoothie Bowl with Greek Yogurt and Honey

Ingredients:

- 1 cup frozen mixed berries
- 1/2 banana
- 1/2 cup plain Greek yogurt
- 1/4 cup almond milk
- 1 tablespoon honey
- Toppings: fresh berries, granola, chia seeds, sliced almonds

Instructions:

1. Blend together the frozen mixed berries, banana, Greek yogurt, almond milk, and honey in a blender. Blend until completely smooth.
2. Fill a bowl halfway with the smoothie mixture.
3. Fresh berries, granola, chia seeds, and sliced almonds go on top.

Green Smoothie Bowl with Kiwi and Hemp Seeds

Ingredients:

- 2 cups baby spinach
- 1 banana
- 1 kiwi, peeled and sliced
- 1/2 avocado
- 1/4 cup almond milk
- 1 tablespoon hemp seeds
- Toppings: sliced kiwi, hemp seeds, sliced almonds

Instructions:

1. In a blender, combine the baby spinach, banana, kiwi, avocado, almond milk, and hemp seeds. Blend until smooth.
2. Pour the smoothie mixture into a bowl.
3. Top with sliced kiwi, hemp seeds, and sliced almonds. Enjoy!

CONCLUSION

As we come to the end of this cookbook, we hope that you have found it to be a valuable resource for your adrenal fatigue relief diet journey. Our goal was to provide you with a range of delicious and nutritious meal options that not only help to reduce stress on your body but also taste great.

Starting with breakfasts that energize and sustain, we offered you an array of nutrient-dense smoothies, nourishing oatmeal bowls, and egg dishes that will give you the perfect start to your day. Moving onto lunches, we provided you with options that will keep you going through your busy day, including wholesome salads and soups, satisfying sandwiches and wraps, and grain and vegetable bowls that are both delicious and satisfying.

For dinner, we have a range of options to restore and recharge your body, including flavorful fish and seafood dishes, comforting meat and poultry dishes, and grilled chicken and veggie skewers with quinoa salad.

Finally, we rounded out the book with snacks that fuel and sustain, including energy bites, roasted chickpeas, and chia pudding.

We understand that making dietary changes can be challenging, but we hope that this cookbook has helped make the transition a little easier for you. Remember, the key to success is to make small changes gradually and consistently. With time, you will start to feel the benefits of a balanced, nutrient-rich diet.

Thank you for choosing this cookbook as your guide to a healthier, happier life. We wish you all the best on your journey towards optimal health and wellness!